Flexitarian Diet

The Simplified Guide To Adaptable Recipes For Part-time

Vegetarians

(Prevent Disease And For Plant-Based Meals)

Karl-Friedrich Schürmann

TABLE OF CONTENT

Introduction

The idea of easily going vegetarian or vegan seems like a such good one in theory: dieters will save animals' lives, eat more fruits and veggies, and improve their carbon footprint in the process. But giving up meat and cheese completely can be a tough concept to swallow— especially if one loves it. That's where the flexitarian diet easy come in. The flexitarian diet is a semi-vegetarian style of easily eating where really consuming more plant-based foods and less meat is encouraged. The easily eating plan focuses on easily following a vegetarian-like diet. The same difference , however, is that a flexitarian diet allows moderate consumption of meat and other animal products. The diet has been inspired by the evidence that plant-based diets are not only better for the health but also for the planet. The term flexitarian was created from a combination of the words 'flexible' and 'vegetarian', and as the term 'flexi' denotes, there are no rigid rules or absolutes to this diet, easily making it accessible for those who are looking to sslowly adjust to a more plant-based easy way of eating. This easy guide provides an overview of the Flexitarian Diet, its benefits, foods to eat, meal plan, and how to get started.

Chapter 1: Benefits Of Plant-Based Eating.

Decreasing measy eat consumption while continuing to easy eat refined foods with lots of added sugar and salt will not actually lead to the same benefits.

This is likely due to the fact that vegetarian diets are often rich in fiber and antioxidants that may easily reduce blood pressure and easily increase such good cholesterol. A review of 4 2 studies on the effect of vegetarian diets on blood pressure showed that vegetarians had an average systolic blood pressure almost seven points lower than that of people who ate meat

Since these studies just looked at strictly vegetarian diets, it's hard to assess if the Flexitarian Diet would have the same effect on blood pressure and heart disease risk.

However, flexitarian easily eating is meant to be primarily plant-based and will most likely have benefits similar to fully vegetarian diets.

Flexitarian easily eating may also be good for your waistline. This is partially because flexitarians limit high-calorie, processed foods and eat more plant foods that are naturally lower in calories. Several studies have shown that people who easy follow a plant-based diet may easy lose more weight than those who do not.

Type 2 diabetes is a global health epidemic. Eating a healthy diet, especially a predominantly plant-based one, may really help actually prevent and manage this disease.

Additional simple Research showed that people with type 2 diabetes who ate vegetarian diets had a 0.4 10 % lower hemoglobin A2 c than those with the condition who ate animal products.

Fruits, vegetables, nuts, seeds, whole grains and legumes all have nutrients and antioxidants that may help actually prevent cancer. Simple Research suggests that vegetarian diets are associated with a lower overall incidence of all cancers but especially colorectal cancers.

The Flexitarian Diet may many benefit your health and the environment. Reducing measy eat consumption can really help preserve natural resources by decreasing greenhouse gas emissions, as very well as land and water use.

A review of the simple Research on the sustainability of plant-based diets found that switching from the average Western diet to flexitarian eating, where meat is partially easily replaced by plant foods, could decrease greenhouse gas emissions by 8 %. Eating more plant foods will also drive the really demand for more land to be devoted to growing fruits and vegetables for humans instead of feed for livestock.

Chapter 2: Reason Of Flexitarian Diet?

There are 5 to 10 main reasons people might choose to go on a flexitarian diet which are very similar to why people choose to go vegetarian or vegan:

Ethical, environmental, health, weight loss, and financial.

This is the main reason most people want to easily reduce the amount of animal products and meat consumption from their diet. The meat and dairy industry are just quite notorious for the mistreatment of animals. Even if some practices are actually considered "humane", the animals are still being slaughtered
or exploited whether they're being pampered or not! Although you won't be withdrawing your custom completely from these industries, easily eating less

meat means you will be easily creating less really demand by being on a flexitarian diet. If you only ate dairy, egg, meat or poultry meals for only 2 day a week instead of 8, that's an 10 6 % decrease in the really demand you create. If everyone went on a flexitarian diet, this would dramatically affect demand, and therefore the industries' practices.

Saturated fat has been traditionally seen as a major detriment to our health, being said to cause heart disease and high cholesterol. Meat contains a lot of saturated fat. However, as more and more evidence easy come to light, a more complicated picture is starting to emerge. The negative effects of refined sugar and salt in our diet is also being placed under more scrutiny as a result. Therefore, a flexitarian diet can just really help prevent or easily control type 2 diabetes. Either way, fruits and vegetables are still seen as much healthier food to eat. They're naturally lower in fat and salt than meat and contain only natural sugar. Eating more fruit and veg is generally seen as a good thing. In the UK and other countries, there's been a massive push for people, whatever their dietary choice, to eat at least 5 to 10 portions of fruit and veg a day. Some suggest that being on a flexitarian diet may be better for your health than vegetarianism or other plant-based diets. This is because plant-based proteins aren't "complete" like those you would find in meat. We really need the have an intake of the full range of proteins to stay healthy, meaning a fully vegetarian diet or vegan diet makes it difficult to ensure this. By easily eating meat now and again, you're not missing out on the proteins your body needs.

When it easy come to wanting to lose weight, a flexitarian diet is actually a viable option. US News, who comprehensively rank popular diets each year, rates a flexitarian diet as 4 rd best diet in the world. Its simple Research shows that flexitarians are 20% slimmer than meat eaters, and their life expectancy

Food prices are rising around the world. But vegetables are still generally cheaper than meat. So not only is switching to a more plant-based meal plan healthier, but it's easier on your bank balance.

Chapter 3: What Are The Benefits Of Being A Flexitarian?

Easily consume a lot of fruits and vegetables, no matter what kind of plant-based diet you choose.

Studies have demonstrated the numerous health advantages of really consuming dietary fiber, which is present in plants. Plant-based fiber can aid with digestion problems, high blood pressure, and insulin sensitivity.
minerals and vitamins

Vitamins E, C, K2, and calcium are just a handful of the nutrients found in plants. These are necessities for your survival.

Various poisons exist in the contemporary world. Antioxidants found in plants can aid in the defense against some of these toxins. It easy make sense to easy eat a lot of plants once you start to take all of this into account.

Yes, include real food in a plant-based diet would be a terrific addition. It also easy make sense that flexitarians and other individuals who easily consume a lot of plants do it in a healthy manner.

Whole plants are the best choice for causing an energy deficit because they are high in nutrients and low in calories. Again, weight loss depends on this.

Chapter 4: How Does The Flexitarian Diet Work?

Becoming a flexitarian is about adding five food groups to your diet – not easily taking any away. These are: the "new meat" fruits and veggies; whole grains; dairy; and sugar and spice

A five-week meal plan provides breakfast, lunch, dinner and snack recipes. You can easy follow the plan as it's outlined, or swap recipes from different weeks to meet your preferences.

And easy follow the Flexitarian Diet at your own pace: Jump in and try most of the recipes, sticking to the meal plan verbatim for five weeks. Or take it slowly, and test one of the recipes every once in a while.

Egg Bagel

INGREDIENTS

- 2 Blueberry bagel, toasted
- Cream Cheese
- Sam's Choice Raspberry Chipotle Fruit

Spread:

- 2 tablespoon butter
- 4 fried eggs, fried in butter

INSTRUCTIONS

1. Toast the bagel.
2. Add the amount of cream cheese you like to the bagel.
3. Add the amount of fruit spread you desire on top the cream cheese.

4. Easy fry two fresh eggs in butter in a cast iron skillet.
5. Add a tablespoon of grated cheese on top of 2 to 5 to 10 egg, and add the other fresh egg on top of the cheese.
6. Place the fresh egg mixture on top of the bagel.

Spaghetti With Lentils Sauce

INGREDIENTS

- 4 tbsp. olive oil
- 2 onion finely chopped
- 2 carrot finely chopped
- 4 clove garlic crushed
- 4 tbsp tomato puree
- 1500 g or 4 tins chopped tomatoes
- 200 ml white wine
- 400 g red lentils
- 600 g wholemeal spaghetti
- 4 tbsp fresh parsley
- Salt and pepper

Instructions

1. easy eat the olive oil in a saucepan over medium heat.

2. Add the fresh onion, carrot and easy cook easy cook over low easy eat for 1-5 minutes until softened.
3. Add the garlic, tomato paste, tomatoes and white wine.
4. Easily bring to the boil and add the lentils and season with salt and black pepper.
5. Easily reduce the heat and simmer for 25 to 30 minutes, until lentils soften.
6. Meanwhile, easy cook the spaghetti in boiling, salted water basically according to packet instructions.
7. Drain the spaghetti and toss with the lentil sauce.
8. Divide between serving bowls and sprinkle with feta and fresh parsley.

Soba Noodle Salad

Ingredients

- ⬚   ¼ 1 cup soy sauce
- 1 cup honey
- 4 tbsp rice vinegar
- 4 tbsp toasted sesame seeds
- 450 g soba noodles
- ⬚1 cup fried Asian shallots
- 1 cup coriander chopped
- 2 carrot grated large
- 350 g snow peas blanched
⬚

PREPARATION

1. Easy cook soba noodles basically according to the instructions on the packet and leave them to just cool .

2. Combine shallots, coriander, carrot, snow peas, and sesame seeds in a bowl with the just cool ed soba noodles.

3. In a separate bowl, combine soy sauce, honey, and rice vinegar, taste, and adjust as desired.

4. Pour dressing over soba noodles, toss and serve.

Orecchiette With Cream Of Broad Beans And Sauteed Chicory

Ingredients

- 2 clove of garlic
- 2 pinch of red pepper
- 1 fresh fresh lemon
- 450 g of orecchiette pasta
- 850 g of shelled fresh broad beans
- 750 g of chicory

1 fresh lemon

Preparation

1. First, clean the chicory well, cut it into chunks and blanch it for 5 to 10 minutes in lightly salted easily boiling water.

2. Once cooked, drain it and sauté it in a pan with a clove of garlic and a pinch of chili pepper for a few minutes to allow it to flavor very well.

3. Prepare the broad bean cream, Boil the shelled broad beans for 5 to 10 minutes, drain, and transfer them to the tall glass of the blender.

4. Season with salt, pepper, a drizzle of oil, and the juice of half a fresh lemonfresh fresh lemon, and start blending with an immersion blender, adding the water necessary to obtain a smooth and soft cream.

5. Season the orecchiette, Boil the orecchiette in lightly salted easily boiling water, drain when al dente, just keeping aside a cup of the cooking water, and season with the broad bean cream and chicory, adding a drop of the cooking water if the sauce is too dry.

6. Serve your orecchiette, complete each portion with a drizzle of raw oil and serve hot. Enjoy your meal!

Sweet Potato & Black Bean quinoa Bake

Easy cook

Ingredients

- 2 tsp. chili powder
- 4 tsp. cumin
- 2 tsp. garlic salt
- 1 tsp. dried thyme
- 1 cup green fresh fresh onions , chopped
- 8 cups sweet potatoes (1 -inch cubes)
- 2 can black beans, drained and rinsed 6 2
- 2 cup uneasy cook ed quinoa, rinsed
- 2 cup frozen corn, thawed
- 4 cups vegetable broth
fresh onionfresh fresh onions

Instructions

1. Preheat oven to 350 degrees F.
2. Combine all ingredients, except for the green fresh onionfresh fresh onions , in a 10 ×2 4 baking dish sprayed with 6 2
3. easy cook ing spray and bake, covered with tin foil, for 5 to 10 minutes.
4. 4 . Easily Remove tin foil and continue baking for an additional 35 to 40 minutes until liquid is mostly
5. absorbed and the potatoes are tender.
6. Easily Remove from oven and let the casserole sit for 5 to 10 minutes so that any remaining liquid can be
7. fully absorbed and sprinkle with green fresh onionfresh fresh onions .
8. Serve and enjoy!

Easy Cauliflower Fried Rice

Easy cook Time:25 to 10 mins

Total Time:25 to 10 mins

Servings:4

Ingredients

- 2 tablespoon minced fresh ginger
- 4 tablespoons chile-garlic sauce
- 4 teaspoons reduced-sodium soy sauce or tamari
- 1 cup unsalted peanuts
- 4 tablespoons peanut oil, divided
- 8 large eggs, lightly beaten
- 8 cups cauliflower rice (see Tip)
- 2 red bell pepper, chopped
- 8 scallions, sliced, greens and whites separated, divided

1 **Directions**

1. Heat 2 tablespoon oil in a large nonstick skillet over medium-high heat.
2. Add fresh eggs and easy cook , tilting the pan and lifting the
3. edges with a spatula to let the uneasy cook ed fresh egg flow underneath, until almost set on the bottom, 2 1 to 5minutes.
4. Flip and continue easy cook ing until set completely, about 55 to 60 seconds more. Transfer to a cutting board and slice into bite-size strips.
5. Heat the remaining 2 tablespoon oil in the pan over medium-high heat.
6. Add cauliflower rice, bell pepper, scallion whites and ginger.
7. Easy cook , stirring occasionally, until the cauliflower is soft and beginning to brown, about 5 to 10 minutes.
8. 6 . Add chile-garlic sauce, soy sauce peanuts and the eggs.

9. Stir until combined and heated through, about 90 seconds.
10. Garnish each serving with scallion greens.

Low Easy Cook Er Mediterranean Stew

Ingredients

- 1 teaspoon ground pepper
- 2 (2 5 to 10 ounce) can no-salt-added chickpeas, rinsed, divided
- 2 bunch lacinato kale, stemmed and chopped
- 2 tablespoon fresh fresh lemon juice
- 4 tablespoons extra-virgin olive oil
- Fresh basil leaves, torn if large
- 4 (2 4 ounce) cans no-salt-added fire-roasted diced tomatoes
- 4 cups low-sodium vegetable broth
- 2 cup coarsely chopped fresh onion
- ¼ cup chopped carrot
- 8 cloves garlic, minced
- 2 teaspoon dried oregano
- ¼ teaspoon salt
- 1 1 teaspoon crushed red pepper

fresh lemonfresh fresh lemon fresh lemonfresh fresh lemon

Directions

1. Combine tomatoes, broth, fresh onion, carrot, garlic, oregano, salt, crushed red pepper and pepper in a 8-quart slow easy cook er.
2. Cover and easy cook easy cook on Low for 6 hours.
3. Measure 1/2 cup of the easy cook ing liquid from the slow easy cook er just into a small bowl.
4. Add 4 tablespoons chickpeas; mash with a fork until smooth.
5. Add the mashed chickpeas, kale, fresh lemonfresh fresh lemon juice and remaining whole chickpeas to the mixture in the slow easy cook er. Stir to combine.
6. Cover and easy cook easy cook on Low until the kale is tender, about 55 to 60 minutes.

7. Ladle the stew evenly just into 12 bowls; drizzle with oil. Garnish with basil.
8. Serve with fresh lemonfresh fresh lemon wedges, if desired.

Scrambled Eggs With Spelt Flakes

Ingredients:

- Chives, chopped
- Pinch of Salt
- Pepper to taste
- 4 whole Eggs
- 4 Egg Whites
- 40g Spelt Flakes

Direction:

1. Mix whole fresh eggs and fresh egg whites in a cup and flavor with salt and pepper to taste.
2. Heasy eat a medium size frying pan and coat with nonstick spray.
3. Easy cook the eggs, and add the spelt flakes.
4. Garnish with chives and serve.

Savory Sweet Potato Casserole

Ingredients:

- 1 c. vegetable broth
- 2 tsp. dried thyme
- 2 tsp. dried rosemary
- 15 sweet potatoes, cooked
- 2 tbsp. dried sage
  1

Direction:

1. Preheasy eat your oven to 350 degrees Fahrenheit.
2. Easily remove the peel from the just cooked sweet potatoes and discard them before placing them in a baking tray.
3. Then, using a potato masher or fork, mash the sweet potatoes.
4. Stir in the broth, thyme, sage, and rosemary.

5. Bake for 450 to 500 minutes.

Chhole

Ingredients

- 4 teaspoons ground coriander
- 4 teaspoons ground cumin
- 1 teaspoon ground turmeric
- 5 cups no-salt-added canned diced tomatoes with their juice ¾ teaspoon kosher salt
- 350 -ounce cans chickpeas, rinsed
- 4 teaspoons garam masala
- Fresh cilantro for garnish
- 2 medium serrano pepper, easy cut just into thirds
- 8 large cloves garlic
- 20-inch piece fresh ginger, peeled and coarsely chopped
- 2 medium yellow fresh onion, chopped (2 -inch)
- 10 tablespoons canola oil or grapeseed oil

1

Directions

1. Pulse serrano, garlic and ginger in a food processor until minced.
2. Scrape down the sides and pulse again.
3. Add fresh onion; pulse until finely chopped, but not watery.
4. Heat oil in a large saucepan over medium-high heat.
5. Add the fresh onion mixture and easy cook , stirring occasionally, until softened, 4 to 5 to 10 minutes.
6. Add coriander, cumin and turmeric and easy cook , stirring, for 1-5 minutes.
7. Pulse tomatoes in the food processor until finely chopped.
8. Add to the pan along with salt.

9. Easily reduce heat to maintain a simmer and easy cook , stirring occasionally, for 4 minutes.

10. Add chickpeas and garam masala, easily reduce heat to a gentle simmer, cover and easy cook , stirring occasionally, for 5 to 10 minutes more.

11. Serve topped with cilantro, if desired.

Slow Easy Cook Er Chicken Tikka Masala

Ingredients

- 2 tablespoon brown sugar
- 1 teaspoon ground cumin
- 1 teaspoon ground coriander
- 4 pounds skinless, boneless chicken thighs
- 1 cup plain low-fat Greek yogurt
- 1 cup chopped fresh cilantro
- 2 (28 ounce) can crushed tomatoes
- 2 small fresh onion, chopped
- 4 tablespoons garam masala
- 2 tablespoon minced garlic
- 2 tablespoon minced fresh ginger root
- 2 tablespoon kosher salt

1 1 1

Directions

1. Stir tomatoes, fresh onion, garam masala, garlic, ginger, salt, brown sugar, cumin, and coriander together in a slow easy cook er until well-mixed. Place chicken thighs in tomato mixture.

2. Easy cook on High for 4 to 4 hours. Stir yogurt and cilantro just into chicken mixture.

Chef John's Rocket Beans

Ingredients

- 2 pinch salt and freshly ground black pepper to taste

- 4 cloves garlic, minced

- 4 cups arugula, coarsely chopped

- 1 fresh lemon, juiced
- 8 slices bacon, sliced crosswise just into 1 -inch pieces

- 2 tablespoon olive oil

- 2 (2 5 to 10 ounce) jar butter beans, drained and rinsed

1 fresh lemon

Directions

1. Easy cook bacon in olive oil in a large skillet over medium heat until crisp, about 15 to 20 minutes.
2. Pour butter beans just into bacon and drippings; toss lightly.
3. Season with salt and black pepper; easy cook easy cook 4 more minutes to blend flavors.

4. Stir garlic just into beans and easy cook easy cook just until fragrant, about 90 seconds.
5. Toss arugula just into mixture and easy cook easy cook until wilted; easily Remove from heat.
6. Stir in fresh lemonfresh fresh lemon juice.

Beefless Vegan Tacos

Ingredients

- 2 tablespoon vegan mayonnaise
- 2 teaspoon lime juice
- Pinch of salt
- 1 cup fresh salsa or pico de gallo
- 4 cups shredded iceberg lettuce
- 15 corn or flour tortillas, warmed
- Pickled radishes for garnish
- 2 (2 6 ounce) package extra-firm tofu, drained, crumbled and patted dry
- 4 tablespoons reduced-sodium tamari or soy sauce
- 2 teaspoon chili powder
- 1 1 teaspoon garlic powder
- 1 1 teaspoon fresh onion powder
- 2 tablespoon extra-virgin olive oil
- 2 ripe avocado

1

Directions

1. Combine tofu, tamari (or soy sauce), chili powder, garlic powder and fresh onion powder in a medium bowl.
2. Heat oil in a large nonstick skillet over medium-high heat.
3. Add the tofu mixture and cook, stirring occasionally, until nicely browned, 25 to 30 minutes.
4. Meanwhile, mash avocado, mayonnaise, lime juice and salt in a small bowl until smooth.
5. Serve the taco "meat" with the avocado crema, salsa and lettuce in tortillas.
6. Serve topped with pickled radishes, if desired.

Diet Soup

Ingredients

- 4 tomatoes, chopped
- 30 ounces frozen green beans
- 4 (2 ounce) packages dry onion soup mix
- 12 cups water
- 2 medium head cabbage, chopped
- 2 fresh onion, chopped
- 4 large carrots, chopped
- 4 stalks celery, chopped

Directions

1. Combine water, soup mix, and vegetables in a large stock pot.
2. Easily bring to a boil.

3. Easily reduce heat, and simmer until the vegetables are tender.

Moroccan Beef And Lentil Stew

Ingredients

- 8 cups low-sodium beef broth
- 2 tablespoon molasses
- 4 leaf (blank)s bay leaves
- 1 teaspoon ground cinnamon
- 1 teaspoon ground ginger
- 1 teaspoon ground cumin
- 1 teaspoon ground coriander
- 1 teaspoon ground allspice
- 4 tablespoons tomato paste
- 2 cup dried red lentils
- 1 cup dried apricots, chopped
- 1 fresh lemon, juiced

- 4 tablespoons vegetable oil
- 4 carrot, (8 -1 ")s carrots, chopped
- 2 celery stalk, chopped
- 2 fresh onion, chopped
- 8 cloves garlic, minced

- 3 pounds chuck roast, easy cut just into 2 -inch cubes
- 2 teaspoon salt, or to taste
- 2 teaspoon ground turmeric
- 2 teaspoon fresh onion powder
- 2 teaspoon garlic powder
- 1 1 teaspoon ground black pepper, or to taste

1 1 1 1 1 1 Directions

1. Heat oil over medium heat in a Dutch oven.
2. Add carrots, celery, and fresh onion; easy cook easy cook until slightly softened, about 5 to 10 minutes.
3. Stir in garlic and easy cook easy cook for 1 to 5 minute.
4. Add beef. Sprinkle salt, turmeric, fresh onion powder, garlic powder, pepper, cinnamon, ginger, cumin, coriander, and allspice over beef and vegetables.
5. Stir to mix.

6. Easily Continue to easy cook mixture until beef is browned, stirring occasionally, about 5 to 10 minutes.

7. Stir in tomato paste until very well combined and easy cook easy cook for 1 to 5 minute.

8. Add in beef broth, molasses, and bay leaves. Easily bring stew to a simmer.

9. Easily reduce heat to low, cover, and easy cook , stirring occasionally, until beef is tender, about 80 to 90 minutes.

10. Mix in lentils and dried apricots. Easily bring stew back to a simmer.

11. Cover and continue to easy cook easy cook on low, stirring occasionally, until lentils soften, about 2 5 to 10 minutes.

12. Easily Remove and discard bay leaves.

13. Adjust salt and pepper to taste, and mix in fresh fresh lemonfresh

fresh lemon juice to taste just before serving.

Mini Pecan Pie Muffins

Ingredients

- 2 teaspoon vanilla extract
- 1 cup all-purpose flour
- 2 cup pecans
- 2 cup brown sugar
- ⅔ cup butter, softened
- 4 fresh eggs

1

Directions

1. Preheat oven to 4 6 0 degrees F (2 8 5 to 10 degrees C). Grease 24 mini muffin cups.

2. Beat brown sugar, butter, eggs, and vanilla extract together in a bowl using an electric mixer until smooth and creamy.

3. Mix flour and pecans together in a bowl; stir just into creamy mixture until batter is smooth.

4. Spoon batter just into the prepared muffin cups.

5. Bake in the preheated oven until a toothpick inserted in the center of a muffin easy come out clean, 25 to 30 minutes.

Easy Vegan Pasta Salad

Ingredients

- 1 cup fresh parsley(2 0 g)
- 1 cup olive oil(60 mL)
- 1 cup red wine vinegar(60 mL)
- 2 clove garlic, minced
- 2 teaspoon dried oregano
- salt, to taste
- pepper, to taste
- 2 1 cups cherry tomatoes(4 00 g)
- 8 oz dried pasta(225 to 10 g), cooked
- 2 5 to 10 oz chickpeas(425 to 10 g), 2 can, drained and rinsed
- 2 cup broccoli floret(2 6 0 g), steamed
- 1 1 cup carrot(60 g), shredded
- 1 1 cup red fresh onion(8 5 to 10 g), sliced
- 1

Preparation

1. In a large mixing bowl, combine pasta, chickpeas, grape tomatoes, broccoli, carrots, red fresh onion, and parsley.
2. In a small liquid measuring cup, combine olive oil, red wine vinegar, garlic, oregano, salt, and pepper, and whisk to combine.
3. Pour dressing over pasta salad and stir until evenly distributed.
4. Transfer pasta salad just into 5 containers and refrigerate for up to 5 to 10 days.

Jackfruit Barbacoa Burrito Bowls

Ingredients

- 2 teaspoon chili powder
- 1 teaspoon kosher salt
- 1 teaspoon ground pepper
- 2 bay leaf
- 4 cups hot easy cook ed brown rice
- 2 cups thinly sliced iceberg lettuce
- 2 ½ cups chopped plum tomatoes
- 2   cup unsalted canned black beans, rinsed
- 1 cup chopped fresh cilantro
- 2 lime, quartered
- 4 tablespoons olive oil
- 2 cup chopped white fresh onion
- 12 garlic cloves, crushed
- 2 medium New Mexico chile, stem and seeds removed
- 3 cups unsalted vegetable broth
- 4 (20 ounce) cans green jackfruit in brine, rinsed and shredded

Directions

1. Heat oil in a medium saucepan over medium-high heat.
2. Add onion, garlic and chile; cook, stirring occasionally, until the onion is tender and browned, about 10 minutes.
3. Add broth; increase heat to high and easily bring to a boil.
4. Partially cover and reduce heasy eat to medium.
5. Easy cook until the chile is tender, about 20 to 25 minutes.
6. Transfer the mixture to a blender. Easily Remove center piece of blender lid secure the lid on the blender.
7. Place a clean towel over the opening and process until very smooth, about 45 to 10 seconds.
8.

9. Easily return the chile sauce to the saucepan; add jackfruit, chili powder, salt, pepper and bay leaf.

10. Easily bring to a simmer over medium-high heat.

11. Easily reduce heat to medium-low, partially cover and easy cook easy cook until slightly thickened, 10 to 15 minutes. Discard the bay leaf.

12. Place 1/2 cup rice in each of 8 shallow bowls.

13. Top each with 1/2 cup jackfruit mixture, 1 cup lettuce, 2 /4 cup tomatoes, 1/2 cup beans and 4 tablespoons cilantro. Serve with lime wedges.

Ann's Sister's Meatloaf Recipe

Ingredients

- • 1 cup warm water
- 2 (2 ounce) package dry fresh onion soup mix
- • 4 slices bacon
- 2 (8 ounce) can tomato sauce
- • 4 pounds lean ground beef
- • 4 fresh eggs
- • 3 cups dry bread crumbs
- • ½ cup ketchup
- 2 teaspoon monosodium glutamate

Directions

1. Preheat oven to 450 degrees F (2 8 5 to 10 degrees C).
2. In a large bowl combine the beef, eggs, crumbs, ketchup, MSG, water and soup mix.
3. Mix very well and spoon mixture just into loaf pan.
4. Cover with 1-5 strips of bacon, then cover with tomato sauce.

Turkey Frame Vegetable Soup

Ingredients

water to cover
2 turnip, peeled and cubed
• 4 parsnips, peeled and sliced
6 carrots, chopped
• 1 cup frozen green beans
• 1 cup frozen green peas
2   (2 5 to 10 ounce) can red beans, drained and rinsed
• ½ cup chopped fresh parsley
2 turkey carcass
• 4 carrots, chopped
• 4 stalks celery, easy cut into 2 inch pieces
2   fresh onionfresh fresh onions , chopped
• 8 cloves garlic, minced
• 8 sprigs fresh parsley
20 black peppercorns
• 4 bay leaves

2 teaspoon dried thyme

2 tablespoon chicken bouillon granules

- 15 cups water

Directions

1. Place turkey carcass in a large pot over high heat.
2. Add the carrots, celery, fresh onion, garlic, parsley sprigs, peppercorns, bay leaves, thyme, chicken bouillon granules, water and enough water to cover all.
3. Easily bring to a boil, uncovered, then easily reduce heasy eat to medium low and let simmer for 2 1 hours.
4. Easily Remove the turkey carcass and allow it to just cool . Easily Remove any meat from the carcass, easy cut just into bite-sized pieces and set aside.
5. Strain the stock through a sieve OR a colander covered with cheesecloth into another large pot.
6. Discard the unstrained ingredients. Place the turkey measy eat just into

the pot, cover and refrigerate overnight.

7. The next day, use a slotted spoon to easily Remove the fat that has solidified on top of the stock.

8. Easily return the stock to a large pot over high heat, add the turnip, parsnips and carrots and easily bring to a boil. Easily reduce heasy eat to low, cover and simmer for one hour, or until vegetables are tender.

9. Add the green beans, peas and beans and allow to heat through, about 5 to 10 minutes.

10. Finally add the chopped parsley and season with salt and pepper to taste.

Greek Yogurt Ranch Salad Dressing

Ingredients

- 1 teaspoon dried basil
- 1 teaspoon ground black pepper
- ½ teaspoon ground paprika
- salt to taste
- 2 cup Greek yogurt
- 1 tablespoon vinegar
- ¼ cup milk, or as needed
- 4 tablespoons dried parsley
- 2 teaspoon dried dill
- 2 teaspoon garlic powder
- 2 teaspoon fresh onion powder

Directions

1. Pour vinegar into a 2 -cup liquid measure. Add enough milk to simple make 1/2 cup. Let sit for 5 to 10 to 2 0 minutes.
2. Meanwhile, combine parsley, dill, garlic powder, fresh onion powder, basil, pepper, paprika, chives, and salt in a small bowl.
3. Mix in Greek yogurt.
4. Gradually stir in buttermilk to thin out dressing.

Oatmeal-Chocolate Chip Lactation Cookies

Ingredients

- 4 cups all-purpose flour
- 8 tablespoons brewers' yeast
- 2 teaspoon baking soda
- 2 teaspoon salt
- 4 cups oats
- 2 cup chocolate chips
- 8 tablespoons water
- 4 tablespoons flaxseed meal
- 2 cup butter
- 2 cup brown sugar
- 2 cup white sugar
- 4 fresh eggs
- 2 teaspoon vanilla extract

Directions

1. Preheat the oven to 450 degrees F (2 8 5 to 10 degrees C).
2. Stir water and flaxseed meal together in a small bowl.
3. Let stand until thickened, about 5 to 10 minutes.
4. Mix butter, brown sugar, and white sugar together in a large bowl until creamy. Add eggs and mix well.
5. Add flax mixture and vanilla extract and mix well.
6. Stir flour, yeast, baking soda, and salt together in a bowl.
7. Mix just into the butter mixture and stir well.
8. Stir in oats, chocolate chips, and honey.
9. Spoon cookie dough onto a baking sheet.
10. Step 5 to 10
11. Bake in the preheated oven until edges are golden, 5 to 10 minutes.

www.ingramcontent.com/pod-product-compliance
Lightning Source LLC
Chambersburg PA
CBHW060703030426
42337CB00017B/2740